Plant-Based Recipes for Busy Lives: Quick and
Delicious Meals for Health-Conscious Individuals

A Comprehensive Guide to Nourishing Your Body with
Easy-to-Prepare Plant-Based Dishes

Author: Nicole Hilliard

Introduction:
-   The concept of plant-based eating and its
    benefits for health and well-being.

Plant-based eating involves consuming primarily
foods derived from plants, such as fruits,
vegetables, whole grains, legumes, nuts, and seeds,
while minimizing or eliminating animal products like
meat, dairy, and eggs. This dietary approach
emphasizes whole, minimally processed foods and
offers numerous health benefits.

Plant-based eating is associated with lower risks of
chronic diseases, including heart disease, diabetes,
and certain cancers. It can help improve heart
health by lowering cholesterol levels and blood
pressure, reduce inflammation in the body, and
support healthy weight management.

Additionally, plant-based diets tend to be rich in
fiber, vitamins, minerals, and antioxidants, which
are essential for overall health and well-being.
They can also promote better digestion, increased
energy levels, and a stronger immune system.

By focusing on plant-based foods, individuals can
enjoy a diverse and delicious array of meals while
nourishing their bodies and supporting a more
sustainable and environmentally friendly food
system.

-   Motivations for adopting a plant-based lifestyle.

There are numerous motivations for adopting a plant-
based lifestyle, and they can vary from person to
person. Some common motivations include:

1. **Health Benefits:** Many people choose a plant-based diet to improve their overall health and well-being. Plant-based eating has been linked to lower risks of chronic diseases such as heart disease, diabetes, obesity, and certain cancers. By focusing on whole, nutrient-dense plant foods, individuals can nourish their bodies with essential vitamins, minerals, fiber, and antioxidants while reducing their intake of saturated fats, cholesterol, and processed foods.

2. **Ethical and Environmental Concerns:** Concerns about animal welfare and environmental sustainability often drive individuals to adopt a plant-based lifestyle. Factory farming practices can be harmful to animals, contributing to their suffering and exploitation. Additionally, animal agriculture is a major contributor to greenhouse gas emissions, deforestation, and water pollution. By choosing plant-based foods, individuals can reduce their environmental footprint and contribute to a more sustainable food system.

3. **Weight Management and Body Composition:** For some people, adopting a plant-based diet can be a strategy for weight management and improving body composition. Plant-based foods tend to be lower in calories and saturated fats while higher in fiber, which can promote feelings of fullness and satiety. By focusing on whole, minimally processed plant foods, individuals can achieve and maintain a healthy weight more easily.

4. **Cultural or Religious Beliefs:** In some cultures and religions, plant-based diets are traditional or prescribed for spiritual or ethical reasons. For example, many Buddhist, Hindu, and Jain traditions advocate for vegetarianism or veganism as a way to practice compassion and non-violence towards all living beings.

5.   **Personal Values and Beliefs:** Individuals may
     adopt a plant-based lifestyle based on personal
     values and beliefs, such as a desire to live in
     alignment with their values of compassion,
     sustainability, or social justice. Choosing
     plant-based foods can be seen as a way to
     express these values and make a positive impact
     on the world.

Overall, there are numerous motivations for adopting
a plant-based lifestyle, and individuals may be
influenced by a combination of health, ethical,
environmental, cultural, and personal factors. By
aligning their dietary choices with their values and
goals, individuals can experience a multitude of
benefits for themselves, animals, and the planet.

-   The purpose and scope of this e-book is to
    provide busy individuals with simple, nutritious,
    and flavorful plant-based recipes that can be
    prepared quickly and easily.

Chapter 1: The Basics of Plant-Based Eating
-   What does it mean to eat a plant-based diet and
    dispelling common misconceptions.

Eating a plant-based diet involves consuming
predominantly foods derived from plants, such as
fruits, vegetables, whole grains, legumes, nuts, and
seeds, while minimizing or excluding animal products
like meat, dairy, eggs, and honey. The focus is on
consuming whole, minimally processed foods in their
natural state, while limiting or avoiding highly
processed and refined products.

Common misconceptions about plant-based diets
include:

1.   **It's Only for Vegans:** While plant-based
     diets are often associated with veganism, they
     are not synonymous. While vegans avoid all
     animal products, including meat, dairy, eggs,
     and honey, plant-based diets can vary in their
     degree of restriction. Some people may follow a
     mostly plant-based diet while occasionally

incorporating small amounts of animal products, while others may eliminate animal products entirely.

2. **It's Nutritionally Incomplete:** Another misconception is that plant-based diets lack essential nutrients and may lead to nutritional deficiencies. However, when properly planned, plant-based diets can provide all the essential nutrients the body needs, including protein, iron, calcium, vitamin B12, omega-3 fatty acids, and more. Whole plant foods are rich in vitamins, minerals, fiber, and antioxidants, which can support overall health and well-being.

3. **It's Expensive:** There's a belief that plant-based diets are more expensive than diets that include meat and dairy. While some specialty plant-based products can be pricey, many plant-based staples such as grains, beans, lentils, fruits, and vegetables are affordable and accessible. Planning meals around these inexpensive ingredients can make plant-based eating cost-effective and budget-friendly.

4. **It's Bland and Boring:** Some people assume that plant-based diets are bland and lack variety and flavor. However, plant-based eating offers a wide array of colorful and flavorful ingredients that can be combined in endless ways to create delicious and satisfying meals. With the right herbs, spices, and cooking techniques, plant-based dishes can be just as flavorful and satisfying as their animal-based counterparts.

By dispelling these misconceptions and understanding what it truly means to eat a plant-based diet, individuals can make informed decisions about their dietary choices and embrace the numerous health, environmental, and ethical benefits that come with plant-based eating.

-   The health benefits of plant-based eating, including improved digestion, weight management, and reduced risk of chronic diseases.

Plant-based eating offers numerous health benefits
across various aspects of well-being, including
improved digestion, weight management, and reduced
risk of chronic diseases. Here's a closer look at
these benefits:

1. **Improved Digestion:** Plant-based diets are
    rich in dietary fiber, which is essential for
    maintaining a healthy digestive system. Fiber
    adds bulk to stool, promotes regular bowel
    movements, and helps prevent constipation.
    Additionally, fiber acts as a prebiotic,
    nourishing beneficial gut bacteria and
    supporting gut health. By consuming a variety of
    fruits, vegetables, whole grains, legumes, nuts,
    and seeds, individuals can optimize their
    digestive health and reduce the risk of
    gastrointestinal issues such as diverticulosis,
    hemorrhoids, and irritable bowel syndrome.

2. **Weight Management:** Plant-based diets are
    naturally lower in calories and saturated fats
    compared to diets that include animal products.
    As a result, they can be effective for weight
    management and promoting a healthy body weight.
    Additionally, plant-based foods tend to be
    higher in fiber, which promotes feelings of
    fullness and satiety, reducing the likelihood of
    overeating. By focusing on whole, minimally
    processed plant foods and incorporating plenty
    of fruits, vegetables, legumes, and whole grains
    into meals, individuals can support their weight
    loss or weight maintenance goals in a
    sustainable and healthful way.

3. **Reduced Risk of Chronic Diseases:** Plant-
    based diets have been associated with a reduced
    risk of chronic diseases, including heart
    disease, diabetes, obesity, hypertension, and
    certain types of cancer. By emphasizing
    nutrient-dense plant foods and minimizing or
    eliminating animal products, individuals can
    reduce their intake of saturated fats,
    cholesterol, and harmful substances found in

processed meats. Plant-based diets are naturally
rich in vitamins, minerals, antioxidants, and
phytonutrients, which have been shown to promote
cardiovascular health, regulate blood sugar
levels, lower blood pressure, and reduce
inflammation. Additionally, plant-based diets
are associated with healthier lipid profiles,
lower levels of LDL cholesterol, and improved
insulin sensitivity, all of which contribute to
a lower risk of chronic diseases over the long
term.

Overall, plant-based eating offers a wealth of
health benefits, including improved digestion,
weight management, and reduced risk of chronic
diseases. By adopting a plant-based diet and
focusing on whole, nutrient-dense plant foods,
individuals can nourish their bodies, support their
health goals, and enhance their overall well-being.

-   Some practical tips for transitioning to a plant-
    based diet, including stocking your pantry with
    essential ingredients and incorporating more
    fruits, vegetables, whole grains, and legumes
    into your meals.

Transitioning to a plant-based diet can be a gradual
process. Here are some practical tips to help ease
the transition:

1. Start gradually: Begin by incorporating more
    plant-based meals into your diet and gradually
    reducing your intake of animal products.

2. Explore plant-based alternatives: Experiment
    with plant-based alternatives to meat, dairy,
    and eggs, such as tofu, tempeh, lentils, beans,
    nuts, and seeds.

3. Focus on whole foods: Base your meals around
    whole, unprocessed plant foods like fruits,
    vegetables, whole grains, legumes, nuts, and
    seeds.

4. Experiment with new recipes: Try out different plant-based recipes to discover new flavors and meal options. There are many online resources, cookbooks, and apps available for inspiration.

5. Incorporate variety: Include a variety of plant foods in your diet to ensure you're getting a wide range of nutrients. Aim to eat a rainbow of fruits and vegetables to maximize nutritional diversity.

6. Plan ahead: Plan your meals and snacks in advance to ensure you have plant-based options available. This can help prevent resorting to convenience foods or falling back on old eating habits.

7. Find plant-based swaps: Look for plant-based alternatives to your favorite dishes, such as veggie burgers, plant-based milk, nut cheeses, and dairy-free desserts.

8. Listen to your body: Pay attention to how your body feels as you transition to a plant-based diet. Make adjustments as needed to ensure you're meeting your nutritional needs and feeling satisfied.

9. Stay informed: Educate yourself about plant-based nutrition to ensure you're getting all the essential nutrients your body needs. Consider consulting with a registered dietitian or nutritionist for personalized guidance.

10. Be patient and kind to yourself: Remember that transitioning to a plant-based diet is a journey, and it's okay to take it one step at a time. Celebrate your progress and focus on the positive changes you're making for your health and the environment.

Chapter 2: Essential Kitchen Tools and Ingredients

Here's a list of essential kitchen tools and ingredients for a plant-based diet:

Kitchen Tools:

1. High-speed blender: Useful for making smoothies, sauces, soups, and nut-based creams.
2. Food processor: Great for chopping, shredding, and blending ingredients for dishes like veggie burgers, hummus, and energy balls.
3. Sharp knives: Essential for chopping fruits, vegetables, and herbs.
4. Vegetable spiralizer: Perfect for turning vegetables like zucchini and carrots into noodles for healthier pasta dishes.
5. Steamer basket: Ideal for steaming vegetables while retaining their nutrients and flavor.
6. Non-stick skillet or frying pan: Useful for cooking tofu, tempeh, and sautéing vegetables without oil.
7. Baking sheets: Essential for roasting vegetables and making plant-based baked goods.
8. Slow cooker or Instant Pot: Convenient for cooking beans, grains, and hearty stews.
9. Mason jars and glass containers: Great for storing homemade sauces, dressings, and leftovers.
10. Nut milk bag: Essential for straining homemade nut milks and making plant-based cheese alternatives.

Essential Ingredients:

1. Whole grains: Quinoa, brown rice, oats, barley, farro, and whole wheat pasta.
2. Legumes: Lentils, chickpeas, black beans, kidney beans, and split peas.
3. Nuts and seeds: Almonds, walnuts, cashews, chia seeds, flaxseeds, and pumpkin seeds.
4. Plant-based proteins: Tofu, tempeh, seitan, and edamame.
5. Fresh fruits and vegetables: A variety of colorful fruits and vegetables to provide a wide range of nutrients.

6. Plant-based milk: Almond, soy, coconut, oat, or
    hemp milk for use in smoothies, cereals, and
    baking.
7. Nutritional yeast: Adds a cheesy flavor to
    dishes and provides a source of vitamin B12.
8. Healthy fats: Avocado, olive oil, coconut oil,
    and nuts for adding flavor and satiety to meals.
9. Herbs and spices: Fresh and dried herbs, spices,
    and seasoning blends to enhance the flavor of
    dishes.
10. Plant-based condiments: Tahini, miso paste, soy
    sauce, balsamic vinegar, and mustard for adding
    flavor to sauces and dressings.

With these kitchen tools and ingredients, you'll
have everything you need to create delicious and
nutritious plant-based meals at home.

-   Essential kitchen tools and equipment that can be
    used for preparing plant-based meals efficiently.

Here are some essential kitchen tools and equipment
specifically geared towards efficiently preparing
plant-based meals:

1. **High-speed blender:** Essential for making
    smoothies, soups, sauces, dressings, and nut-
    based creams.

2. **Food processor:** Perfect for chopping,
    shredding, and blending ingredients for dishes
    like veggie burgers, hummus, and energy balls.

3. **Sharp knives:** Essential for chopping,
    slicing, and dicing fruits, vegetables, and
    herbs.

4. **Vegetable spiralizer:** Ideal for turning
    vegetables like zucchini, carrots, and sweet
    potatoes into noodles for pasta dishes or
    salads.

5. **Steamer basket:** Useful for steaming
    vegetables while retaining their nutrients and
    flavor.

6. **Non-stick skillet or frying pan:** Handy for cooking tofu, tempeh, and sautéing vegetables without oil.

7. **Baking sheets:** Essential for roasting vegetables, making plant-based baked goods, and preparing crispy tofu or chickpeas.

8. **Large pot and saucepans:** Necessary for cooking grains, beans, lentils, and preparing soups, stews, and pasta dishes.

9. **Silicone baking mats or parchment paper:** Useful for lining baking sheets to prevent sticking when roasting vegetables or baking.

10. **Salad spinner:** Great for washing and drying leafy greens and herbs efficiently.

11. **Mason jars and glass containers:** Ideal for storing homemade sauces, dressings, leftovers, and prepped ingredients.

12. **Nut milk bag:** Essential for straining homemade nut milks and making plant-based cheese alternatives.

13. **Microplane grater/zester:** Handy for grating citrus zest, ginger, garlic, and hard cheeses (if you're using vegan alternatives).

14. **Measuring cups and spoons:** Essential for accurately measuring ingredients for recipes, especially when baking.

15. **Tongs and spatulas:** Useful for flipping, stirring, and serving various ingredients during cooking.

These tools and equipment will help streamline your plant-based meal preparation process and make it more efficient and enjoyable.

-   Key ingredients that can be used in plant-based
    cooking, such as grains, beans, nuts, seeds,
    fruits, and vegetables.

Here are some key ingredients used in plant-based
cooking, categorized by food group:

Grains:
1. Quinoa
2. Brown rice
3. Oats
4. Barley
5. Farro
6. Bulgur
7. Millet
8. Buckwheat
9. Whole wheat pasta
10. Couscous (whole wheat or gluten-free)

Beans and Legumes:
1. Lentils (green, brown, red, or black)
2. Chickpeas (garbanzo beans)
3. Black beans
4. Kidney beans
5. Cannellini beans
6. Navy beans
7. Pinto beans
8. Split peas
9. Black-eyed peas
10. Edamame (young soybeans)

Nuts and Seeds:
1. Almonds
2. Walnuts
3. Cashews
4. Pistachios
5. Pecans
6. Hazelnuts
7. Sunflower seeds
8. Pumpkin seeds (pepitas)
9. Chia seeds
10. Flaxseeds

Fruits:
1. Apples

2. Bananas
3. Oranges
4. Berries (strawberries, blueberries, raspberries, blackberries)
5. Mangoes
6. Pineapple
7. Kiwi
8. Grapes
9. Pears
10. Avocado

Vegetables:
1. Leafy greens (spinach, kale, Swiss chard, arugula)
2. Broccoli
3. Cauliflower
4. Carrots
5. Bell peppers (red, yellow, green)
6. Tomatoes
7. Cucumbers
8. Zucchini
9. Sweet potatoes
10. Mushrooms

These ingredients form the foundation of a plant-based diet and can be used in countless combinations to create delicious and nutritious meals. They provide a wide range of essential nutrients, including protein, fiber, vitamins, minerals, and healthy fats, making them integral to a balanced and healthy eating pattern.

- Tips for sourcing high-quality, organic, and seasonal ingredients on a budget.

Here are some tips for sourcing high-quality, organic, and seasonal ingredients on a budget:

1. **Shop at local farmers' markets:** Farmers' markets often offer a variety of fresh, locally grown produce at competitive prices. You can find organic and seasonal fruits and vegetables while supporting local farmers.

2. **Join a community-supported agriculture (CSA)
    program:** CSA programs allow you to purchase a
    share of a local farm's harvest in advance,
    typically at a discounted rate. You'll receive a
    box of fresh, seasonal produce each week or
    month, depending on the program.

3. **Buy in bulk:** Purchasing staples like grains,
    beans, nuts, and seeds in bulk can help you save
    money in the long run. Look for bulk bins at
    health food stores or buy online from wholesale
    retailers.

4. **Grow your own produce:** If you have space,
    consider starting a small vegetable garden or
    growing herbs indoors. It's a cost-effective way
    to access fresh, organic produce, and you'll
    have control over the growing process.

5. **Opt for frozen produce:** Frozen fruits and
    vegetables are often more affordable than fresh
    and can be just as nutritious. Plus, they're
    convenient and have a longer shelf life,
    reducing food waste.

6. **Compare prices and look for sales:** Take the
    time to compare prices at different grocery
    stores and look for sales and promotions on
    organic and seasonal items. You can also sign up
    for newsletters or loyalty programs to receive
    discounts.

7. **Use apps and websites for discounts:** Utilize
    apps and websites that offer discounts, coupons,
    or cashback rewards for organic and natural
    products. Some examples include Ibotta, Checkout
    51, and Thrive Market.

8. **Focus on in-season produce:** Buying fruits
    and vegetables that are in season can help lower
    costs since they're more abundant and typically
    cheaper. Plus, seasonal produce tends to be
    fresher and tastier.

9.   **Prioritize certain organic items:** If buying
     everything organic isn't feasible due to budget
     constraints, prioritize purchasing organic
     versions of the "Dirty Dozen" â€” a list of
     produce items that tend to have higher pesticide
     residues. Items on this list include
     strawberries, spinach, kale, apples, and grapes.

10.   **Consider alternative sources:** Explore
      alternative sources for organic and seasonal
      ingredients, such as local co-ops, online
      farmers' markets, or food rescue organizations
      that offer surplus produce at discounted
      prices.

By implementing these strategies, you can make it
more affordable to incorporate high-quality,
organic, and seasonal ingredients into your plant-
based diet.

Chapter 3: Breakfast Recipes

- A collection of quick and nutritious plant-based
   breakfast recipes.

Here are 20 quick and nutritious plant-based
breakfast recipes with variations and substitutions
to accommodate different dietary preferences:

1.   **Avocado Toast:**
     - Variation: Top with sliced radishes,
        microgreens, and a sprinkle of Everything But
        The Bagel seasoning.
     - Substitution: Use gluten-free bread for a
        gluten-free option.

2.   **Smoothie Bowl:**
     - Variation: Add a spoonful of nut butter or a
        handful of spinach for extra creaminess and
        nutrition.
     - Substitution: Use almond milk, coconut milk,
        or soy milk as a base.

3.   **Overnight Oats:**

   - Variation: Mix in cocoa powder and chopped
     nuts for a chocolatey twist.
   - Substitution: Use maple syrup or agave syrup
     as a sweetener instead of honey.

4. **Chia Seed Pudding:**
   - Variation: Layer with mashed berries or fruit
     compote for added flavor.
   - Substitution: Use coconut milk or almond milk
     instead of regular milk.

5. **Tofu Scramble:**
   - Variation: Add diced bell peppers, mushrooms,
     or sun-dried tomatoes for extra flavor.
   - Substitution: Use black salt (kala namak) for
     an eggy flavor.

6. **Banana Pancakes:**
   - Variation: Mix in blueberries or chocolate
     chips for added sweetness.
   - Substitution: Use mashed sweet potato or
     pumpkin puree instead of banana.

7. **Quinoa Breakfast Bowl:**
   - Variation: Stir in a spoonful of nut butter
     and sliced bananas for a protein boost.
   - Substitution: Use cooked amaranth or buckwheat
     instead of quinoa.

8. **Veggie Breakfast Burrito:**
   - Variation: Add sliced avocado, salsa verde, or
     hot sauce for extra flavor.
   - Substitution: Use corn tortillas for a gluten-
     free option.

9. **Greek Yogurt Parfait:**
   - Variation: Layer with homemade granola and a
     drizzle of date syrup or honey.
   - Substitution: Use coconut yogurt or almond
     yogurt for a dairy-free option.

10. **Sweet Potato Toast:**
   - Variation: Top with almond butter, sliced
     strawberries, and a sprinkle of hemp seeds.

        - Substitution: Use butternut squash slices
          instead of sweet potato.

11.   **Berry Breakfast Bowl:**
        - Variation: Mix in a spoonful of hemp seeds or
          ground flaxseeds for added omega-3s.
        - Substitution: Use frozen mixed berries if
          fresh ones are not available.

12.   **Peanut Butter Banana Smoothie:**
        - Variation: Blend in a handful of spinach or
          kale for an extra nutritional boost.
        - Substitution: Use sunflower seed butter or
          almond butter instead of peanut butter.

13.   **Fruit Salad:**
        - Variation: Drizzle with a mixture of lime
          juice and maple syrup for a refreshing citrus
          flavor.
        - Substitution: Use seasonal fruits like
          apples, pears, or citrus fruits.

14.   **Coconut Yogurt Bowl:**
        - Variation: Sprinkle with toasted coconut
          flakes and cacao nibs for added crunch.
        - Substitution: Use cashew yogurt or soy yogurt
          instead of coconut yogurt.

15.   **Hummus Toast:**
        - Variation: Top with sliced cherry tomatoes,
          fresh basil leaves, and a drizzle of balsamic
          glaze.
        - Substitution: Use gluten-free hummus and
          bread for a gluten-free option.

16.   **Energy Balls:**
        - Variation: Roll in shredded coconut or
          crushed nuts for different textures.
        - Substitution: Use date paste or mashed
          bananas as a natural sweetener.

17.   **Savory Breakfast Muffins:**
        - Variation: Add nutritional yeast and chopped
          olives for a cheesy Mediterranean flavor.

- Substitution: Use chickpea flour or almond
  flour for a gluten-free option.

18. **Green Smoothie:**
  - Variation: Add a scoop of plant-based protein
    powder for an extra protein boost.
  - Substitution: Use kale, spinach, or Swiss
    chard as the leafy green base.

19. **Oatmeal Raisin Cookies:**
  - Variation: Stir in shredded carrots and
    ground cinnamon for a carrot cake-inspired
    cookie.
  - Substitution: Use raisins, dried cranberries,
    or chopped dates instead of raisins.

20. **Breakfast Tacos:**
  - Variation: Top with sliced avocado, pickled
    jalapenos, and a squeeze of lime juice for a
    zesty kick.
  - Substitution: Use gluten-free tortillas or
    lettuce wraps for a low-carb option.

These variations and substitutions offer flexibility
to accommodate different taste preferences, dietary
needs, and ingredient availability while still
providing quick and nutritious plant-based breakfast
options.

Chapter 4: Lunch and Dinner Recipes
- A variety of satisfying plant-based lunch and
  dinner options.

21. satisfying plant-based lunch and dinner options,
    including salads, soups, sandwiches, wraps,
    stir-fries, and grain bowls, all of which can be
    prepared in under 30 minutes:

1. **Mediterranean Chickpea Salad:**
  - Combine chickpeas, cherry tomatoes, cucumber,
    red onion, Kalamata olives, and parsley. Dress
    with olive oil, lemon juice, garlic, and
    oregano.

2. **Coconut Curry Lentil Soup:**

   - Sautée onions, garlic, ginger, and curry
     paste. Add red lentils, coconut milk,
     vegetable broth, and diced vegetables. Simmer
     until lentils are tender.

3. **Veggie Stir-Fry with Tofu:**
   - Stir-fry tofu, bell peppers, broccoli,
     carrots, and snap peas in a sauce made from
     soy sauce, garlic, ginger, and sesame oil.
     Serve over rice or noodles.

4. **Caprese Sandwich:**
   - Layer sliced tomatoes, fresh basil leaves, and
     vegan mozzarella cheese on whole grain bread.
     Drizzle with balsamic glaze and season with
     salt and pepper.

5. **Quinoa Black Bean Salad Bowl:**
   - Mix cooked quinoa with black beans, corn,
     diced bell peppers, avocado, and cilantro.
     Dress with lime juice, olive oil, cumin, and
     chili powder.

6. **Vegan Caesar Salad:**
   - Toss chopped romaine lettuce with vegan Caesar
     dressing, croutons, and vegan Parmesan cheese.
     Top with grilled tofu or chickpeas for added
     protein.

7. **Thai Peanut Noodle Bowl:**
   - Cook rice noodles according to package
     instructions. Toss with shredded cabbage,
     carrots, bell peppers, and a homemade peanut
     sauce. Garnish with chopped peanuts and
     cilantro.

8. **Sweet Potato and Black Bean Quesadillas:**
   - Mash cooked sweet potatoes and mix with black
     beans, diced red onion, and spices. Spread
     mixture onto tortillas, top with vegan cheese,
     and cook until crispy.

9. **Mushroom and Spinach Pasta:**
   - Sautée sliced mushrooms and garlic in olive
     oil. Add cooked pasta, baby spinach, lemon

zest, and red pepper flakes. Toss until
   spinach wilts.

10.   **Falafel Wrap:**
   -   Stuff whole wheat wraps with homemade or
       store-bought falafel, shredded lettuce,
       tomatoes, cucumbers, and tahini sauce.

11.   **Mexican Quinoa Salad Bowl:**
   -   Mix cooked quinoa with black beans, corn,
       diced tomatoes, avocado, cilantro, and lime
       juice. Top with salsa and sliced jalapenos
       for extra flavor.

12.   **Miso Vegetable Soup:**
   -   Simmer miso paste, vegetable broth, tofu,
       mushrooms, bok choy, and green onions. Serve
       garnished with sesame seeds and nori strips.

13.   **Grilled Portobello Mushroom Burgers:**
   -   Marinate portobello mushroom caps in balsamic
       vinegar, garlic, and olive oil. Grill until
       tender and serve on whole grain buns with
       lettuce, tomato, and avocado.

14.   **Chickpea Shawarma Bowl:**
   -   Toss roasted chickpeas with quinoa,
       tabbouleh, cucumber slices, and tahini sauce.
       Sprinkle with sumac for an extra burst of
       flavor.

15.   **Vegetable Pad Thai:**
   -   Stir-fry rice noodles with tofu, bean
       sprouts, bell peppers, carrots, and green
       onions in a tangy tamarind sauce. Garnish
       with crushed peanuts and lime wedges.

16.   **Greek Salad Pita Pockets:**
   -   Fill whole wheat pita pockets with chopped
       cucumber, tomatoes, red onion, Kalamata
       olives, and vegan feta cheese. Drizzle with
       olive oil and red wine vinegar.

17.   **Sesame Ginger Tofu Stir-Fry:**

- Sauté tofu, broccoli, bell peppers, snow
  peas, and carrots in a sesame ginger sauce.
  Serve over brown rice or quinoa.

18. **Black Bean and Corn Tacos:**
    - Fill corn tortillas with black beans, corn,
    diced avocado, shredded lettuce, and salsa.
    Top with cilantro and a squeeze of lime
    juice.

19. **Lentil Spinach Dal:**
    - Simmer lentils with onion, garlic, ginger,
    tomato, spinach, and spices like cumin,
    turmeric, and coriander. Serve over rice or
    with naan bread.

20. **Mediterranean Veggie Wrap:**
    - Wrap hummus, roasted vegetables (like
    eggplant, zucchini, and red peppers),
    spinach, and olives in a whole grain
    tortilla. Drizzle with balsamic glaze and
    enjoy.

These flavorful plant-based recipes are not only
quick to prepare but also packed with nutrients,
making them perfect for busy weekdays or evenings.

Chapter 5: Snacks and Appetizers

Here are 20 wholesome plant-based snacks and
appetizers, along with an emphasis on balanced
snacking and portion control for maintaining energy
levels throughout the day:

1. **Hummus and Veggie Sticks:** Pair homemade or
    store-bought hummus with sliced carrots, celery,
    bell peppers, cucumber, and cherry tomatoes for
    a satisfying and nutritious snack.

2. **Guacamole and Whole Grain Crackers:** Enjoy
    mashed avocado mixed with lime juice, diced
    tomatoes, onions, and cilantro, served with
    whole grain crackers for a flavorful and filling
    snack.

3. **Roasted Chickpeas:** Season cooked chickpeas
    with olive oil, salt, and spices like paprika,
    garlic powder, or cumin. Roast in the oven until
    crispy for a crunchy and protein-rich snack.

4. **Energy Balls:** Blend dates, nuts, seeds, and
    cocoa powder in a food processor. Roll into
    bite-sized balls and refrigerate for a
    convenient and energy-boosting snack.

5. **Avocado Toast:** Spread mashed avocado onto
    whole grain toast and top with sliced tomatoes,
    a sprinkle of sea salt, and a drizzle of olive
    oil for a delicious and nutrient-dense snack.

6. **Vegetable Sushi Rolls:** Fill nori sheets with
    cooked brown rice, avocado slices, cucumber
    sticks, and shredded carrots. Roll tightly and
    slice into bite-sized pieces for a refreshing
    and portable snack.

7. **Stuffed Mini Bell Peppers:** Fill halved mini
    bell peppers with hummus, guacamole, or a
    mixture of quinoa and black beans for a colorful
    and satisfying snack.

8. **Greek Yogurt with Berries:** Enjoy plant-based
    yogurt topped with fresh berries and a drizzle
    of honey or maple syrup for a creamy and
    antioxidant-rich snack.

9. **Edamame with Sea Salt:** Boil edamame pods in
    salted water until tender. Drain and sprinkle
    with sea salt for a protein-packed and
    satisfying snack.

10. **Nut Butter Apple Slices:** Spread almond
    butter, peanut butter, or cashew butter onto
    apple slices and sprinkle with cinnamon or
    granola for a crunchy and satisfying snack.

11. **Caprese Skewers:** Thread cherry tomatoes,
    basil leaves, and vegan mozzarella balls onto
    skewers. Drizzle with balsamic glaze and

sprinkle with salt and pepper for a flavorful appetizer.

12. **Cucumber Bites:** Top cucumber slices with hummus, salsa, or guacamole for a refreshing and low-calorie snack.

13. **Trail Mix:** Combine nuts, seeds, dried fruit, and dark chocolate chips for a balanced and portable snack that provides a mix of healthy fats, protein, and carbohydrates.

14. **Stuffed Dates:** Remove pits from dates and fill with almond butter, tahini, or vegan cream cheese. Sprinkle with crushed nuts or coconut flakes for a sweet and satisfying snack.

15. **Rice Cake with Avocado and Tomato:** Spread mashed avocado onto a rice cake and top with sliced tomatoes and a sprinkle of nutritional yeast or hemp seeds for a light and crunchy snack.

16. **Chia Pudding:** Mix chia seeds with plant-based milk and sweetener of choice. Let sit in the fridge until thickened, then top with fresh fruit, nuts, or granola for a nutritious and filling snack.

17. **Veggie Spring Rolls:** Fill rice paper wrappers with shredded lettuce, carrots, cucumber, bell peppers, and fresh herbs. Serve with a side of peanut sauce or sweet chili sauce for dipping.

18. **Spinach and Artichoke Dip with Whole Grain Pita Chips:** Enjoy a creamy and flavorful spinach and artichoke dip with whole grain pita chips for a satisfying and crowd-pleasing appetizer.

19. **Stuffed Mushrooms:** Fill mushroom caps with a mixture of breadcrumbs, spinach, garlic, and vegan cheese. Bake until golden and bubbly for a delicious and savory snack.

20.   **Chickpea Salad Lettuce Wraps:** Mix mashed
       chickpeas with diced vegetables, lemon juice,
       and herbs. Spoon into lettuce leaves and roll
       up for a light and refreshing snack.

Balanced snacking involves choosing snacks that
provide a combination of macronutrients
(carbohydrates, protein, and fats) to help keep you
satisfied and energized throughout the day. It's
also important to practice portion control and
listen to your body's hunger and fullness cues.
Enjoying snacks mindfully can help prevent
overeating and support overall health and well-
being.

Chapter 6: Desserts and Treats

Here are some guilt-free plant-based desserts and
treats that will satisfy your sweet tooth without
relying on refined sugars or artificial ingredients.
These recipes use natural sweeteners and whole-food
ingredients for delicious and wholesome indulgence:

1.   **Banana Nice Cream:**
     - Blend frozen bananas with a splash of plant-
       based milk until smooth and creamy. Add
       toppings like berries, nuts, and coconut
       flakes for extra flavor and texture.

2.   **Date-Sweetened Energy Bars:**
     - Blend dates, nuts, seeds, and dried fruit in a
       food processor until sticky. Press into a pan
       and refrigerate until firm. Cut into bars for
       a nutritious and portable snack.

3.   **Raw Chocolate Avocado Mousse:**
     - Blend ripe avocados, cocoa powder, dates, and
       a splash of almond milk until smooth and
       creamy. Chill in the fridge before serving for
       a decadent and healthy dessert.

4.   **Coconut Date Balls:**
     - Blend dates, shredded coconut, and a pinch of
       sea salt in a food processor until combined.

Roll into balls and coat in more shredded
coconut for a naturally sweet and satisfying
treat.

5. **Baked Apple Crisp:**
   - Slice apples and toss with cinnamon, nutmeg,
   and a drizzle of maple syrup. Top with a
   mixture of rolled oats, chopped nuts, coconut
   oil, and a touch of coconut sugar. Bake until
   golden and bubbly.

6. **Chia Seed Pudding Parfait:**
   - Mix chia seeds with plant-based milk and
   sweetener of choice. Let sit in the fridge
   until thickened, then layer with fresh fruit,
   nuts, and granola for a nutritious and
   delicious parfait.

7. **Almond Butter Cups:**
   - Melt dairy-free chocolate chips and pour a
   small amount into mini muffin liners. Top with
   a spoonful of almond butter and cover with
   more melted chocolate. Chill until set for a
   homemade version of this classic treat.

8. **Frozen Grape Popsicles:**
   - Skewer grapes and freeze until firm for a
   refreshing and naturally sweet frozen treat.

9. **Berry Crumble Bars:**
   - Mix oats, almond flour, coconut oil, and maple
   syrup to form a crumbly dough. Press half of
   the mixture into a pan, top with mixed
   berries, and sprinkle with the remaining
   crumble. Bake until golden brown.

10. **Peanut Butter Banana Bites:**
    - Spread peanut butter onto banana slices and
    sandwich together. Dip in melted dark
    chocolate and sprinkle with chopped nuts or
    coconut flakes. Chill until chocolate sets
    for a satisfying and sweet snack.

11. **Mango Coconut Popsicles:**

- Blend fresh mango with coconut milk and a
  touch of agave syrup until smooth. Pour into
  popsicle molds and freeze until solid for a
  tropical and refreshing treat.

12. **No-Bake Lemon Coconut Bars:**
  - Mix shredded coconut, almond flour, lemon
  zest, and maple syrup until well combined.
  Press into a pan and refrigerate until firm.
  Cut into bars and enjoy the zesty flavor
  without any guilt.

13. **Cacao Date Truffles:**
  - Blend dates, cacao powder, and a pinch of
  salt in a food processor until a sticky dough
  forms. Roll into balls and coat in crushed
  nuts or coconut flakes for a rich and
  chocolatey treat.

14. **Pumpkin Spice Energy Bites:**
  - Mix rolled oats, pumpkin puree, almond
  butter, maple syrup, and pumpkin spice until
  well combined. Roll into balls and
  refrigerate until firm for a seasonal and
  satisfying snack.

15. **Frozen Banana Pops:**
  - Insert popsicle sticks into peeled bananas
  and dip in melted dark chocolate. Roll in
  chopped nuts, coconut flakes, or dried fruit
  and freeze until chocolate sets for a fun and
  customizable frozen treat.

16. **Raw Walnut Brownies:**
  - Blend walnuts, dates, cocoa powder, and a
  pinch of sea salt in a food processor until
  sticky. Press into a pan and refrigerate
  until firm. Cut into squares for a rich and
  fudgy dessert.

17. **Blueberry Oat Bars:**
  - Mix oats, almond flour, mashed banana, and
  blueberries until well combined. Press into a
  pan and bake until golden brown for a
  wholesome and fruity snack.

18. **Homemade Mango Sorbet:**
     - Blend frozen mango chunks with a splash of
       coconut water until smooth and creamy. Serve
       immediately for a refreshing and naturally
       sweet dessert.

19. **Chocolate Covered Strawberries:**
     - Dip fresh strawberries into melted dairy-free
       chocolate and place on a lined baking sheet.
       Chill in the fridge until chocolate sets for
       an elegant and decadent treat.

20. **Cinnamon Maple Roasted Almonds:**
     - Toss raw almonds with maple syrup, cinnamon,
       and a pinch of salt. Roast in the oven until
       golden and crunchy for a sweet and satisfying
       snack.

These guilt-free plant-based desserts and treats are
perfect for satisfying your sweet cravings while
providing nourishment and natural sweetness from
wholesome ingredients. Enjoy them in moderation as
part of a balanced and healthy lifestyle.

Chapter 7: Meal Planning and Batch Cooking

Certainly! Here are some practical tips for meal
planning and batch cooking to streamline your plant-
based meal preparation process:

1. **Set Aside Time for Planning:** Dedicate a
    specific day each week to plan your meals for
    the upcoming week. This can help you stay
    organized and ensure you have all the
    ingredients you need on hand.

2. **Create a Weekly Meal Plan:** Use a meal
    planning template or app to outline your meals
    for breakfast, lunch, dinner, and snacks.
    Include a variety of plant-based recipes to
    ensure you're getting a balanced diet.

3. **Batch Cook Staples:** Identify recipes that
    can be batch-cooked in advance, such as grains

(rice, quinoa, etc.), beans, lentils, roasted vegetables, and sauces. Cook large batches and portion them out for easy meal assembly throughout the week.

4. **Prep Ingredients in Advance:** Wash, chop, and portion out fruits and vegetables ahead of time to save time during meal preparation. Store them in airtight containers or reusable bags in the fridge for easy access.

5. **Utilize Freezer-Friendly Meals:** Prepare freezer-friendly meals like soups, stews, casseroles, and veggie burgers in large batches. Portion them out into individual servings and freeze for quick and convenient meals later on.

6. **Plan for Leftovers:** Incorporate meals that make good leftovers into your meal plan, such as hearty salads, grain bowls, and pasta dishes. Cook extra portions to enjoy for lunch or dinner the next day.

7. **Stock Up on Staples:** Keep your pantry stocked with essential plant-based ingredients like grains, beans, lentils, canned tomatoes, coconut milk, nuts, seeds, and spices. This makes it easier to throw together quick and nutritious meals.

8. **Be Flexible:** Allow for flexibility in your meal plan to accommodate changes in schedule or unexpected events. Have a few backup meals or simple recipes on hand for busy days when you don't have time to cook.

9. **Minimize Food Waste:** Plan meals that use overlapping ingredients to minimize food waste. Use up leftover ingredients in creative ways, such as adding them to soups, salads, or stir-fries.

10. **Rotate Recipes:** Create a repertoire of favorite plant-based recipes and rotate them regularly. This can help simplify meal planning

and grocery shopping while ensuring you're still enjoying a variety of flavors and nutrients.

Sample Plant-Based Meal Plan Template:

Monday:
- Breakfast: Overnight oats with mixed berries and almond butter.
- Lunch: Chickpea salad wraps with whole grain tortillas and a side of carrot sticks.
- Dinner: Lentil and vegetable curry served over brown rice.
- Snack: Apple slices with peanut butter.

Tuesday:
- Breakfast: Green smoothie made with spinach, banana, mango, and plant-based protein powder.
- Lunch: Quinoa and black bean salad bowl with avocado, corn, tomatoes, and cilantro.
- Dinner: Veggie stir-fry with tofu, broccoli, bell peppers, and snap peas served over quinoa.
- Snack: Homemade trail mix with nuts, seeds, and dried fruit.

Wednesday:
- Breakfast: Whole grain toast topped with mashed avocado, sliced tomatoes, and Everything But The Bagel seasoning.
- Lunch: Sweet potato and black bean quesadillas with a side of salsa and mixed greens.
- Dinner: Roasted vegetable and chickpea buddha bowls with tahini dressing.
- Snack: Hummus and veggie sticks (carrots, cucumbers, bell peppers).

Thursday:
- Breakfast: Chia seed pudding with almond milk, mixed berries, and a sprinkle of hemp seeds.
- Lunch: Greek salad pita pockets filled with chopped cucumbers, tomatoes, red onion, olives, and vegan feta cheese.
- Dinner: Mushroom and spinach pasta with garlic, lemon zest, and nutritional yeast.

- Snack: Frozen banana pops dipped in dark
  chocolate and chopped nuts.

Friday:
- Breakfast: Smoothie bowl topped with granola,
  sliced banana, and coconut flakes.
- Lunch: Falafel wraps with homemade falafel,
  shredded lettuce, tomatoes, cucumbers, and tahini
  sauce.
- Dinner: Lentil soup with carrots, celery, onions,
  and kale served with crusty whole grain bread.
- Snack: Date-sweetened energy balls made with
  oats, dates, nuts, and cinnamon.

By following these tips and incorporating a meal
plan like the sample template provided, you can
streamline your plant-based meal preparation
process, save time, and reduce food waste while
enjoying delicious and nutritious meals throughout
the week.

Conclusion:

Key Takeaways from "Plant-Based Recipes for Busy
Lives":

1. **Quick and Delicious Meals:** The e-book
    provides a wide range of plant-based recipes
    that are quick and easy to prepare, perfect for
    individuals with busy lifestyles.

2. **Nutritious and Balanced:** Each recipe is
    designed to be both delicious and nutritionally
    balanced, ensuring that you can nourish your
    body with wholesome plant-based ingredients.

3. **Variety and Flavor:** Embrace the diverse
    flavors and ingredients of plant-based eating,
    from hearty grain bowls to refreshing salads and
    satisfying desserts.

4. **Meal Planning and Batch Cooking:** Learn how
    to streamline your meal preparation process with
    practical tips for meal planning, batch cooking,
    and minimizing food waste.

5. **Health-Conscious Choices:** By choosing plant-
    based meals, you can support your health and
    well-being while reducing your environmental
    footprint and promoting sustainability.

6. **Flexibility and Adaptability:** Plant-based
    eating is flexible and adaptable, allowing you
    to customize recipes to suit your taste
    preferences, dietary needs, and lifestyle.

Encouragement to Embrace Plant-Based Eating:

-   Embrace plant-based eating as a sustainable and
    nourishing lifestyle choice that can benefit both
    your health and the planet.
-   Experiment with new ingredients, flavors, and
    cooking techniques to expand your culinary
    repertoire and discover the joy of plant-based
    cooking.
-   Prioritize whole, minimally processed foods and
    incorporate plenty of fruits, vegetables,
    legumes, whole grains, nuts, and seeds into your
    meals.
-   Start small by incorporating plant-based meals
    into your routine and gradually increasing their
    frequency over time.
-   Celebrate the abundance and variety of plant-
    based foods and the positive impact they can have
    on your health, the environment, and animal
    welfare.

Overall, "Plant-Based Recipes for Busy Lives"
encourages readers to embrace plant-based eating as
a sustainable, nourishing, and delicious lifestyle
choice that can benefit both individuals and the
planet.

Certainly! Here are additional resources for further
exploration of plant-based cooking and living:

1. **Websites:**
    -   **Minimalist Baker:** Offers simple and
        delicious plant-based recipes with minimal
        ingredients and easy-to-follow instructions.

   - **Oh She Glows:** Features a variety of vegan
     recipes, meal plans, and cooking tips from
     cookbook author Angela Liddon.
   - **Forks Over Knives:** Provides evidence-based
     articles, recipes, meal plans, and cooking
     courses focused on a whole-food, plant-based
     lifestyle.
   - **The Happy Pear:** Run by twin brothers Dave
     and Steve, this website offers plant-based
     recipes, meal plans, cooking videos, and
     wellness tips.
   - **Nourish Atelier:** Provides plant-based
     recipes and cooking tutorials, with a focus on
     seasonal and sustainable eating.

2. **Cookbooks:**
   - **"Thug Kitchen: Eat Like You Give a F*ck" by
     Thug Kitchen:** Offers a humorous and
     irreverent approach to plant-based cooking,
     with flavorful recipes for every meal.
   - **"The Oh She Glows Cookbook" by Angela
     Liddon:** Features over 100 vegan recipes,
     including crowd-pleasing classics and
     inventive plant-based dishes.
   - **"Plant-Based on a Budget" by Toni Okamoto:**
     Provides affordable and accessible plant-based
     recipes, meal plans, and shopping tips for
     those on a budget.
   - **"Isa Does It: Amazingly Easy, Wildly
     Delicious Vegan Recipes for Every Day of the
     Week" by Isa Chandra Moskowitz:** Offers 150
     recipes for quick and easy plant-based meals,
     with a focus on flavor and simplicity.
   - **"Power Plates: 100 Nutritionally Balanced,
     One-Dish Vegan Meals" by Gena Hamshaw:**
     Provides balanced and satisfying plant-based
     meals designed to nourish and energize.

3. **Online Communities:**
   - **r/PlantBasedDiet:** A subreddit dedicated to
     discussions, recipes, and support for those
     following a plant-based diet.
   - **Happy Herbivore Community:** Offers forums,
     meal plans, and resources for those interested
     in plant-based eating and living.

- **Veggie Boards:** An online community where users can share recipes, tips, and support for vegetarian and vegan lifestyles.
- **Plant-Based Cooking Facebook Group:** A community of plant-based cooking enthusiasts sharing recipes, cooking tips, and inspiration.
- **Instagram:** Follow plant-based chefs, bloggers, and influencers for recipe ideas, cooking inspiration, and tips for living a plant-based lifestyle.

These resources offer a wealth of information, inspiration, and support for anyone interested in exploring plant-based cooking and living. Whether you're a beginner or a seasoned plant-based eater, there's something for everyone to discover and enjoy!

Appendix:

Glossary of Terms:

1. **Plant-Based Diet:** A diet that emphasizes whole, minimally processed plant foods such as fruits, vegetables, grains, legumes, nuts, and seeds, while minimizing or eliminating animal products.

2. **Whole Foods:** Foods that are minimally processed and close to their natural state, such as fruits, vegetables, whole grains, legumes, nuts, and seeds.

3. **Minimally Processed:** Foods that have undergone minimal processing and retain most of their natural nutrients and fiber.

4. **Nutritional Yeast:** A deactivated yeast often used as a cheese substitute in plant-based cooking. It is rich in B vitamins, including B12, and has a cheesy flavor.

5. **Tofu:** A versatile soy-based protein made from curdled soy milk. It comes in various

textures, including silken, soft, firm, and
extra-firm, and can be used in a variety of
dishes.

6. **Tempeh:** A fermented soybean product that is
    high in protein and fiber. It has a nutty flavor
    and firm texture, making it a popular meat
    substitute in plant-based cooking.

7. **Seitan:** Also known as wheat gluten or wheat
    meat, seitan is made from wheat gluten and has a
    chewy texture similar to meat. It is high in
    protein and commonly used in vegetarian and
    vegan dishes.

8. **Legumes:** A category of plants that includes
    beans, lentils, peas, and chickpeas. Legumes are
    rich in protein, fiber, vitamins, and minerals,
    making them a staple in plant-based diets.

9. **Grains:** Cereal crops such as rice, quinoa,
    barley, oats, and wheat. Grains are a good
    source of carbohydrates, fiber, and various
    nutrients and are often used as the base of
    plant-based meals.

10. **Nuts and Seeds:** Nutrient-dense foods that
    provide healthy fats, protein, fiber, vitamins,
    and minerals. Common examples include almonds,
    walnuts, chia seeds, flaxseeds, and hemp seeds.

11. **Nutritional Information:**
    - Provides information about the nutritional
      content of key ingredients, including
      calories, macronutrients (carbohydrates,
      protein, fat), vitamins, and minerals.
    - Helps individuals make informed dietary
      choices and ensure they are meeting their
      nutritional needs.

12. **Conversion Charts:**
    - Provides conversions for common measurements
      used in cooking, such as cups to grams,
      teaspoons to milliliters, and ounces to
      grams.

- Helps ensure accuracy and consistency when following recipes, especially when using different measurement systems or kitchen tools.

- Weekly meal planning template
ï¿¼

- Grocery shopping list Template

ï¿¼